Table of Contents

What is the Autoimmune Protocol Diet?

A healthy immune system is designed to produce antibodies that attack foreign or harmful cells in your body. However, in people with autoimmune disorders, the immune system tends to produce antibodies that, rather than fight infections, attack healthy cells and tissues. This can result in a range of symptoms, including joint pain, fatigue, abdominal pain, diarrhea, brain fog, and tissue and nerve damage. A few examples of autoimmune disorders include rheumatoid arthritis, lupus, IBD, type 1 diabetes, and psoriasis. Autoimmune diseases are thought to be caused by a variety of factors, including genetic propensity, infection, stress, inflammation, and medication use.

Also, some research suggests that, in susceptible individuals, damage to the gut barrier can lead to increased intestinal permeability, also known as "leaky gut," which may trigger the development of certain autoimmune diseases. Certain foods are believed to possibly increase the gut's permeability, thereby increasing your likelihood of leaky gut. The AIP diet focuses on eliminating these foods and replacing them with health-promoting, nutrient-dense foods that are thought to help heal the gut, and ultimately, reduce inflammation and symptoms of autoimmune diseases. It also removes certain ingredients like gluten, which may cause abnormal immune responses in susceptible individuals. While experts believe that a leaky gut may be a plausible explanation for the inflammation experienced by people with autoimmune disorders, they warn that the current research makes it impossible to confirm a cause-and-effect relationship between the two.Therefore, more research is needed before strong conclusions can be made. The Autoimmune Protocol (AIP) diet is purported to reduce inflammation, pain, and other symptoms experienced by people with autoimmune disorders by healing their leaky gut and removing potentially problematic ingredients from their diet. The AIP is an elimination diet, so it involves not eating certain types of food for several weeks at a time and carefully noting any effects on health. Researchers have described the AIP diet as an extension of the paleo diet. A person usually eats lean proteins, vegetables, fruits, nuts, and seeds. The AIP diet focuses on foods rich in vitamins and other nutrients. A person following it will not eat anything with added sugar or other additives that can trigger an autoimmune response. A person should adhere to the diet strictly for a few weeks, then slowly reintroduce the eliminated foods and take careful note of any reaction. A reaction, such as a surge in symptoms, can indicate that they should exclude that food in the long term. If you have a metabolic or digestive health condition, you may need to avoid foods that trigger allergies or cause your condition to flare up with symptoms. For some autoimmune diseases, you have to eliminate foods or ingredients completely. Otherwise, you won't experience relief from your symptoms, and your gut cannot heal.

The AIP diet is also called the hunter-gatherer diet because it is based on foods available during the Paleolithic time period. Any foods that emerged 10,000 years ago with the invention of farming are excluded from the AIP diet for autoimmune disorders.

Examples of autoimmune disorders include:

- Sjogren's
- Type 1 Diabetes
- Rheumatoid Arthritis
- Celiac Disease
- Polycystic Ovarian Syndrome (PCOS)
- Hashimoto's Disease
- Psoriatic Arthritis
- Adrenal fatigue
- Multiple Sclerosis
- Reoccurring viral infections
- Low immunity
- Lupus

Understanding your digestive system. Your gut has what scientists call a microbiota, populations of microbial species that live in your body. Most of these bacteria, fungi, and viruses live symbiotically with us, causing no harm. You have anywhere from 10-100 microbial cells at any given time. Things we eat, medicines we take, and our feelings impact our microbiota. When the balance is disturbed, it can trigger an illness to develop or a health condition to flare up. Autoimmune diseases are considered inflammatory since they flood your guy with white blood cells to heal the disturbance. The AIP diet places emphasis on identifying and removing the foods that cause inflammation in your gut. When your digestive system stays inflamed, it cannot function properly. This may lead to:

- Poor absorption of nutrients
- Vomiting or diarrhea
- Stomach pain and tenderness
- Cramping

Why the AIP diet?

The theory behind the AIP diet is that avoiding gut-irritating foods and eating nutrient-rich ones will reduce inflammation. One hypothesis about how autoimmune conditions begin is called the leaky gut theory. It states that if there is a problem with the bacterial composition of a person's gut, environmental triggers of inflammation such as toxins and viruses can breach the gut wall and access other parts of the body. Supporters of this theory say that eating the right foods may help prevent symptoms of inflammation, although many experts are skeptical. Many proponents of the leaky gut theory believe that the AIP diet can help prevent the immune system from attacking tissues and reduce the symptoms of autoimmune diseases.

How does it work?

The AIP diet resembles the paleo diet, both in the types of foods allowed and avoided, as well as in the phases that comprise it. Due to their similarities, many consider the AIP diet an extension of the paleo diet though AIP may be seen as a stricter version of it.

The AIP diet consists of two main phases.

The elimination phase

The first phase is an elimination phase that involves the removal of foods and medications believed to cause gut inflammation, imbalances between levels of good and bad bacteria in the gut, or an immune response. During this phase, foods like grains, legumes, nuts, seeds, nightshade vegetables, eggs, and dairy are completely avoided. Tobacco, alcohol, coffee, oils, food additives, refined and processed sugars, and certain medications, such as non-steroidal anti-inflammatory drugs (NSAIDs) should also be avoided

Examples of NSAIDs include ibuprofen, naproxen, diclofenac, and high dose aspirin.

On the other hand, this phase encourages the consumption of fresh, nutrient-dense foods, minimally processed meat, fermented foods, and bone broth. It also emphasizes the improvement of lifestyle factors, such as stress, sleep, and physical activity. The length of the elimination phase of the diet varies, as it's typically maintained until a person feels a noticeable reduction in symptoms. On average, most people maintain this phase for 30–90 days, but some may notice improvements as early as within the first 3 weeks.

The reintroduction phase

Once a measurable improvement in symptoms and overall well-being occurs, the reintroduction phase can begin. During this phase, the avoided foods are gradually reintroduced into the diet, one at a time, based on the person's tolerance.

The goal of this phase is to identify which foods contribute to a person's symptoms and reintroduce all foods that don't cause any symptoms while continuing to avoid those that do. This allows for the widest dietary variety a person can tolerate.

During this phase, foods should be reintroduced one at a time, allowing for a period of 5–7 days before reintroducing a different food. This allows a person enough time to notice if any of their symptoms reappear before continuing the reintroduction process. Foods that are well tolerated can be added back into the diet, while those that trigger symptoms should continue to be avoided. Keep in mind that your food tolerance may change over time.

As such, you may want to repeat the reintroduction test for foods that initially failed the test every once in a while.

Step-by-step reintroduction protocol

Here's a step-by-step approach to reintroducing foods that were avoided during the elimination phase of the AIP diet.

Step 1. Choose one food to reintroduce. Plan to consume this food a few times per day on the testing day, then avoid it completely for 5–6 days.

Step 2. Eat a small amount, such as 1 teaspoon of the food, and wait 15 minutes to see if you have a reaction.

Step 3. If you experience any symptoms, end the test and avoid this food. If you have no symptoms, eat a slightly larger portion, such as 1 1/2 tablespoons, of the same food and monitor how you feel for 2–3 hours.

Step 4. If you experience any symptoms over this period, end the test and avoid this food. If no symptoms occur, eat a normal portion of the same food and avoid it for 5–6 days without reintroducing any other foods.

Step 5. If you experience no symptoms for 5–6 days, you may reincorporate the tested food into your diet, and repeat this 5-step reintroduction process with a new food.

It's best to avoid reintroducing foods under circumstances that tend to increase inflammation and make it difficult to interpret results. These include during an infection, following a poor night's sleep, when feeling unusually stressed, or following a strenuous workout. Additionally, it's sometimes recommended to reintroduce foods in a particular order. For example, when reintroducing dairy, choose dairy products with the lowest lactose concentration to reintroduce first, such as ghee or fermented dairy products. The AIP diet first eliminates any foods that may trigger symptoms for a few weeks. Each is then reintroduced individually so that only those that don't trigger symptoms can ultimately be added back into the diet.

Foods to eat and avoid

The AIP diet has strict recommendations regarding which foods to eat or avoid during its elimination phase

Foods to avoid

Grains: rice, wheat, oats, barley, rye, etc., as well as foods derived from them, such as pasta, bread, and breakfast cereals

Legumes: lentils, beans, peas, peanuts, etc., as well as foods derived from them, such as tofu, tempeh, mock meats, or peanut butter

Nightshade vegetables: eggplants, peppers, potatoes, tomatoes, tomatillos, etc., as well as spices derived from nightshade vegetables, such as paprika

Eggs: whole eggs, egg whites, or foods containing these ingredients

Dairy: cow's, goat's, or sheep's milk, as well as foods derived from these milks, such as cream, cheese, butter, or ghee; dairy-based protein powders or other supplements should also be avoided

Nuts and seeds: all nuts and seeds and foods derived from them, such as flours, butter, or oils; also includes cocoa and seed-based spices, such as coriander, cumin, anise, fennel, fenugreek, mustard, and nutmeg

Certain beverages: alcohol and coffee

Processed vegetable oils: canola, rapeseed, corn, cottonseed, palm kernel, safflower, soybean, or sunflower oils

Refined or processed sugars: cane or beet sugar, corn syrup, brown rice syrup, and barley malt syrup; also includes sweets, soda, candy, frozen desserts, and chocolate, which may contain these ingredients

Food additives and artificial sweeteners: trans fats, food colorings, emulsifiers, and thickeners, as well as artificial sweeteners, such as stevia, mannitol, and xylitol

Some AIP protocols further recommend avoiding all fruit both fresh or dried during the elimination phase. Others allow the inclusion of 10–40 grams of fructose per day, which amounts to around 1–2 portions of fruit per day.

Although not specified in all AIP protocols, some also suggest avoiding algae, such as spirulina or chlorella, during the elimination phase, as this type of sea vegetable may also stimulate an immune response

Foods to eat

Vegetables: a variety of vegetables except for nightshade vegetables and algae, which should be avoided

Fresh fruit: a variety of fresh fruit, in moderation

Tubers: sweet potatoes, taro, yams, as well as Jerusalem or Chinese artichokes

Minimally processed meat: wild game, fish, seafood, organ meat, and poultry; meats should be wild, grass-fed or pasture-raised, whenever possible

Fermented, probiotic-rich foods: nondairy-based fermented food, such as kombucha, kimchi, sauerkraut, pickles, and coconut kefir; probiotic supplements may also be consumed

Minimally processed vegetable oils: olive oil, avocado oil, or coconut oil

Herbs and spices: as long as they're not derived from a seed

Vinegars: balsamic, apple cider, and red wine vinegar, as long as they're free of added sugars

Natural sweeteners: maple syrup and honey, in moderation

Certain teas: green and black tea at average intakes of up to 3–4 cups per day

Bone broth

Despite being allowed, some protocols further recommend that you moderate your intake of salt, saturated and omega-6 fats, natural sugars, such as honey or maple syrup, as well as coconut-based foods.

Depending on the AIP protocol at hand, small amounts of fruit may also be allowed. This usually amounts to a maximum intake of 10–40 grams of fructose per day, or the equivalent of about 1–2 portions of fresh fruit.

Some protocols further suggest moderating your intake of high glycemic fruits and vegetables, including dried fruit, sweet potatoes, and plantain. The glycemic index (GI) is a system used to rank foods on a scale of 0 to 100, based on how much they will increase blood sugar levels, compared with white bread. High glycemic fruits and vegetables are those ranked 70 or above on the GI scale. The AIP diet typically consists of minimally processed, nutrient-dense foods. The lists above specify which foods to eat or avoid during the elimination phase of the AIP diet.

Does the AIP diet work?

Though research on the AIP diet is limited, some evidence suggests that it may reduce inflammation and symptoms of certain autoimmune diseases. Few clinical studies have looked into the effectiveness of the AIP diet — in general or as a means of managing any specific autoimmune disease. In 2017, some researchers found that eliminating certain foods as part of the AIP diet improved symptoms of inflammatory bowel disease. In a 2019 study, 17 female participants aged 20–45 with

Hashimoto's thyroiditis, another autoimmune disease, followed the AIP diet as part of a 10-week health coaching program.Tests showed no changes, but the participants reported a reduction in symptoms and an improvement in their quality of life. The authors suggested that the AIP diet, as part of a wider treatment program, could help people with the condition. Some scientific evidence suggests a link between gut health and inflammatory disease. A growing body of research, for example, indicates that there may be a link between bacterial growth in the gut and inflammatory and autoimmune diseases, such as Crohn's disease. Other studies suggest that the composition of gut bacteria may trigger immune and inflammatory reactions in other parts of the body. In addition, researchers have noted that inflammation affects how well the gut wall functions and that food allergies can make it more porous. This could indicate a link between problems with the gut wall and autoimmune diseases, and confirming it will require further studies. Supporting claims that the AIP diet can reduce symptoms of other autoimmune diseases will require more research.

Health Benefits

May help heal a leaky gut

People with autoimmune diseases often have a leaky gut, and experts believe there may be a link between the inflammation they experience and the permeability of their gut. A healthy gut typically has a low permeability. This allows it to act as a good barrier and prevent food and waste remains from leaking into the bloodstream. However, a highly permeable or leaky gut allows foreign particles to crossover into the bloodstream, in turn, possibly causing inflammation.In parallel, there's growing evidence that the foods you eat can influence your gut's immunity and function, and in some cases, possibly even reduce the degree of inflammation you experience. hypothesis entertained by researchers is that by helping heal leaky gut, the AIP diet may help reduce the degree of inflammation a person experiences. Although scientific evidence is currently limited, a handful of studies suggests that the AIP diet may help reduce inflammation or symptoms caused by it, at least among a subset of people with certain autoimmune disorders.However, more research is needed to specifically understand the exact ways in which the AIP diet may help, as well as the precise circumstances under which it may do so

May reduce inflammation and symptoms of some autoimmune disorders

To date, the AIP diet has been tested in a small group of people and yielded seemingly positive results. For instance, in a recent 11-week study in 15 people with IBD on an AIP diet, participants reported experiencing significantly fewer IBD-related symptoms by the end of the study. However, no significant changes in markers of inflammation were observed. Similarly, a small study had people with IBD follow the AIP diet for 11 weeks.

Participants reported significant improvements in bowel frequency, stress, and the ability to perform leisure or sport activities as early as 3 weeks into the study. In another study, 16 women with Hashimoto's thyroiditis, an autoimmune disorder affecting the thyroid gland, followed the AIP diet for 10 weeks. By the end of the study, inflammation and disease-related symptoms decreased by 29% and 68%, respectively. Participants also reported significant improvements in their quality of life, despite there being no significant differences in their measures of thyroid function. Although promising, studies remain small and few. Also, to date, they have only been performed on a small subset of people with autoimmune disorders. Therefore, more research is needed before strong conclusions can be made.

The AIP diet may help reduce gut permeability and inflammation in people with autoimmune diseases. Small studies report beneficial effects in people with IBD and Hashimoto's thyroiditis, but more research is needed to confirm these benefits.

Possible downsides

The AIP diet is considered an elimination diet, which makes it very restrictive and potentially hard to follow for some, especially in its elimination phase. The elimination phase of this diet can also make it difficult for people to eat in social situations, such as at a restaurant or friend's house, increasing the risk of social isolation. It's also important to note

that there's no guarantee that this diet
will reduce inflammation or disease-
related symptoms in all people with
autoimmune disorders. However, those
who experience a reduction in symptoms
following this diet may be reticent to
progress to the reintroduction phase, for
fear it may bring the symptoms back. This
could become problematic, as remaining
in the elimination phase can make it
difficult to meet your daily nutrient
requirements. Therefore, remaining in
this phase for too long may increase your
risk of developing nutrient deficiencies, as
well as poor health over time. This is why
the reintroduction phase is crucial and
should not be skipped. If you're
experiencing difficulties getting started
with the reintroduction phase, consider
reaching out to a registered dietitian or
other medical professional

knowledgeable about the AIP diet for personalized guidance.

The AIP diet may not work for everyone, and its elimination phase is very restrictive. This can make this diet isolating and hard to follow. It may also lead to a high risk of nutrient deficiencies if its reintroduction phase is avoided for too long.

Pros and cons

Pros of the AIP Diet

The AIP diet can improve your autoimmune disease symptoms. Living with an autoimmune disease can be very difficult. You don't know when you'll have a flare-up that affects your day-to-day life.

With control of your diet, you can help manage your symptoms better and live life with less worry.

The AIP diet can help you lose weight. Since the AIP diet eliminates a lot of unhealthy foods, you can lose weight efficiently. If you've struggled to lose weight on other diets, the AIP might work. Keep in mind that when you begin to reintroduce foods, you'll want to do so in moderation to maintain your weight loss.

Cons of the AIP Diet

The AIP diet is very restrictive. While knowing exactly what you can eat helps you meal plan, it may also be difficult to follow. If you go out to eat, there may not be something on the menu that fits your diet restrictions. If other people in your home are not following the AIP diet, you must be mindful of which foods in your house are safe and which ones aren't.

You may miss out on vital nutrients. Cutting out whole grains means eliminating an excellent source of fiber from your diet. Cutting out dairy means removing your main source of calcium for building strong bones. Make a list of acceptable foods that fill these needs in your diet and be sure to incorporate them regularly.

Should you try it?

The AIP diet is designed to help reduce inflammation, pain, or other symptoms caused by autoimmune diseases. As such, it may work best for people with autoimmune diseases, such as lupus, IBD, celiac disease, or rheumatoid arthritis. Autoimmune diseases cannot be cured, but their symptoms may be managed. The AIP diet aims to help you do so by helping you identify which foods may be triggering your specific symptoms. Evidence regarding the efficacy of this diet is currently limited to people with IBD and Hashimoto's disease. However, based on the way in which this diet is believed to function, people with other autoimmune diseases may benefit from it, too.

There are currently few downsides to giving this diet a try, especially when performed under the supervision of a dietitian or other medical professional. Seeking professional guidance prior to giving the AIP diet a try will help you better pinpoint which foods may be causing your specific symptoms, as well as ensure that you continue to meet your nutrient requirements as best as possible throughout all phases of this diet. The AIP diet may reduce the severity of symptoms associated with various autoimmune diseases. However, it may be difficult to implement on your own, which is why guidance from a dietitian or medical professional is strongly recommended.

AIP Breakfast Bowl

Ingredients

- 1 large broccoli crown
- 1 small head of cauliflower
- 1 small vidalia onion
- 2 garlic cloves
- 1 cup water (or bone broth)
- 1 1/2 teaspoon pink Himalaya salt, divided
- 2 slices bacon
- 6 jumbo shrimp
- 1 tablespoon coconut aminos
- 1 teaspoon dried cilantro or parsley

Instructions

- Chop up broccoli, cauliflower, onion and garlic. Combine in your pressure cooker.
- Add in the water and 1/2 tsp salt. Close and set to the vegetable setting, or on low for 7 minutes..
- Put your bacon on a sheet pan and then in the oven, set to 375F.
- In a bowl toss together the shrimp and remaining salt. Set aside.
- When the oven reaches 375F, check on the bacon. When it's almost done, add the shrimp to the same sheet pan. Roast it all together for 5 minutes. Open the oven, give the sheet pan a shake. Roast another 2-3 minutes.
- By now the pressure cooker should be done with the vegetables. Add all the veggies and half the liquid in to a

blender, and puree until smooth. You can add the remaining liquid if you want it less thick. Taste it, add in more salt as needed.

- Serve 2 cups of the vegetable puree in a bowl, you will have a lot left over! Save it.
- Remove shrimp and bacon from oven. Chop up shrimp and bacon carefully and serve over vegetable puree.
- Drizzle bacon fat over your dish, then coconut aminos and lastly cilantro. Dig in!

AIP Breakfast Stack

Ingredients

- 4 slices AIP-friendly bacon
- 1 pound ground turkey
- 1 medium zucchini, grated coarsely
- 1/4 teaspoon dried sage
- couple of pinches of salt
- coconut oil (if needed)
- 4 large flat mushrooms, stalks removed
- 2 medium avocados, stone and skin removed
- juice of one small lemon
- rocket or watercress leaves

Instructions

- Fry bacon in a large, dry skillet over medium heat until crispy. Set bacon aside. Leave fat in pan.
- In a bowl, blend the turkey, zucchini, sage and a pinch of salt. Form into 6 patties. refrigerate 2 for a snack later; cook 4 now.
- If there's not enough bacon fat in the skillet, add a little coconut oil. Cook patties 5-6 minutes per side. Check they are fully cooked throughout and then remove from pan and set aside.
- Add mushrooms to skillet along with a splash of water. Cook for a few minutes each side, until they turn golden. Turn off the heat.
- Quickly mash the avocado flesh together with a pinch of salt and the lemon juice.

- To assemble: place the upturned mushroom on a plate and arrange a small tangle of the watercress or rocket leaves on top. Place the turkey and zucchini patty on top of that and finish with a spoonful of guacamole and a slice of bacon. Eat while hot.

Autoimmune Healing Bowls

Ingredients

- 1 cup mashed garlic cauliflower
- 2 cups arugula, packed
- 4 oz cooked chicken breast
- 1/4 avocado
- 1 tsp lemon juice
- 1 tsp olive oil
- 1/4 tsp turmeric

- 1/8 tsp salt

Instructions

- Warm the mashed garlic cauliflower and the cooked chicken breast in whatever way is easiest for you. I typically have these pre-cooked, and just need to warm them up in the oven. My recommendation is to put them on a plate, cover with foil, and place in the oven at 300°.
- While the cauliflower and chicken are warming, heat a saucepan over medium heat. Add a small amount of water to the pan, then add the arugula and toss just until wilted. Turn off pan.
- Cut the avocado into slices lengthwise and remove skin.

- Remove plate from oven once cauliflower and chicken are warm.
- Fill a bowl with the mashed garlic cauliflower. Top with the chicken, wilted arugula, and avocado.
- Combine the olive oil, lemon juice, turmeric, and salt in a bowl and whisk.

Nightshade-Free AIP Curry

Ingredients

- 1 (15-ounce) can full-fat coconut milk, see note*
- 2 Tbsp minced ginger
- 3 cloves garlic, minced, optional
- 2 large carrots, peeled and sliced
- 1 large crown broccoli, chopped into florets

- 1 yellow squash, chopped
- 1 large boneless skinless chicken breast
- 2 Tbsp coconut aminos
- 1 tsp ground turmeric
- 1/2 tsp ground cinnamon
- 1/2 tsp sea salt, to taste
- 1 lime, cut into wedges
- 1/2 cup fresh basil, chopped for serving

Instructions

- Pour 1/4 cup of the coconut milk into a large skillet and heat to medium. Add the ginger and garlic, and cook until fragrant, about 2 to 3 minutes.
- Add the carrots and broccoli and cover. Cook, stirring occasionally,

until veggies have softened but are still al dente, about 3 minutes.

- Heat a small amount of coconut oil or avocado oil in a separate skillet over medium heat. Add the chopped chicken. Brown the chicken, stirring occasionally, until a great deal of liquid comes out, about 5 minutes. You don't need to cook the chicken all the way through - you're simply cooking out the liquid. Strain the liquid from the chicken, then add the chicken to the skillet with the vegetables.

- Add the remaining ingredients (including the rest of the coconut milk) except for the lime wedges and basil to the skillet with the vegetables and chicken. Stir well and bring to a full boil, then reduce the heat to a simmer and cover. Cook 15 minutes, then uncover and continue cooking another 8 to 10 minutes, until curry has thickened and chicken is cooked through.

- Taste curry for flavor and add sea salt to taste. Serve with choice of cauliflower rice or other riced vegetables or regular rice. Garnish with lime wedges and basil.

Notes

*Be sure to get coconut milk without any added gums/emulsifiers to keep this recipe AIP

AIP Coffee

Ingredients

- 1 tbsp roasted dandelion root
- 1 tbsp roasted chicory powder
- 1 tbsp carob powder
- 1 date, pitted
- 3 cups water

Instructions

- Combine all ingredients in a small saucepan and bring to a boil.
- Lower heat and allow the mixture to simmer for 5 minutes.
- Remove from heat, strain and serve.

AIP Flatbread Recipe

INGREDIENTS

- 1 13.5 oz can Coconut Milk OR 1.5 cups homemade Coconut Milk or Tigernut Milk
- 3/4 cup Cassava Flour OR Tigernut Flour
- 3/4 cup Tapioca Flour OR Arrowroot Powder
- 1 Pinch of Sea Salt

INSTRUCTIONS

- Preheat a small nonstick pan over medium heat.
- Mix all of the ingredients into a bowl. If using tigernut flour, really make sure all of the lumps are

broken apart (it really likes to clump). Make sure the batter is somewhat runny, you don't want it really thick. Add water or more milk if necessary.

- Pour enough batter into the pan to cover the bottom of the pan + about 1/8-1/4 inch thick. These are a tad bit thicker than crepes.
- Cook for 3-4 minutes per side, adjusting the time up above 4 min if the batter doesn't look completely dry when you flip it, and adjust the time down if you get too many brown or black spots. Black or brown spots are totally fine, just don't want to burn these!
- You'll notice that the cooking time will get less as you continue to cook the breads, since the pan gets hotter. If the bread is gummy inside it needs

to be cooked longer. (This all sounds kind of fussy and complicated but trust me, you'll figure it out after a few – it's just different pans, cassava flours, coconut milks, amount of heat, etc all makes it a little bit different for everyone).

Honey Ginger Salmon

Ingredients

- 1 2" knob ginger
- 2 garlic cloves
- 4 T coconut aminos
- 1 T honey (OR sub with maple syrup)
- 4 T olive oil
- 1 lemon
- 4 salmon fillets, 4-6 oz each

Instructions

- Preheat oven to 425 F.
- Peel and grate ginger for 1T and chop 2 cloves garlic.
- Whisk together the following: 1T grated ginger + 2 chopped garlic cloves + 4T coconut aminos + 1T honey (or maple syrup) + 4T olive oil + 1T lemon juice from 1 lemon.
- Marinate salmon for 30 minutes.
- Remove salmon from marinade and bake for 15-18 minutes or cooked through/flaky.

BACON & 'EGGS' AIP BREAKFAST

INGREDIENTS

- 6 slices bacon thick-cut, uncured
- 1 head cauliflower cut into (4) 1" thick cauliflower steaks
- 2 tablespoons water
- 1 teaspoon liquid coconut aminos
- ⅛ teaspoon ground turmeric

INSTRUCTIONS

- Preheat the oven to 400 degrees F.
- Line a baking sheet with parchment paper.
- Gently lie the bacon slices down flat, followed by the cauliflower steaks. Ensure everything lies flat on the sheet.

- In a small bowl, whisk together the water, liquid coconut aminos, and turmeric.
- Gently brush the mixture over the cauliflower steaks.
- Place the sheet pan in the oven and bake for 20 minutes.
- Remove, serve, and enjoy.

Easy AIP Chicken Stir Fry

INGREDIENTS

- 2 tbsp olive oil use sesame oil if you aren't AIP for added flavor
- 1 cup carrots thinly sliced
- 1 cup onion sliced
- 1 cup AIP Stir Fry Sauce optional, see notes
- 2 Boneless chicken thighs

- 1 tbsp chopped cilantro optional

INSTRUCTIONS

- Heat 1 tablespoon of oil in a saute pan over medium heat.
- Place the chicken in the pan and brown 4 minutes on each side.
- Remove the chicken from the pan and set aside to cool, then slice into strips
- Heat the remaining tablespoon of oil in a pan over high heat then add the vegetables
- Sautee the vegetables until they begin to soften (about 3-5 minutes)
- Add the sliced chicken and pre-made stir fry sauce to the pan and continue to cook another 2-3 minutes

- Plate the stir fry and top with cilantro for garnish

EASY AIP SMOOTHIE

Ingredients

- 1 cup frozen strawberries
- 1 cup frozen pineapple
- 1 cup coconut milk

INSTRUCTIONS

- Add all ingredients to a blender.
- Blend on high until smooth and creamy.
- Pour into a glass and enjoy!

Pumpkin Spice Coconut Breakfast Porridge

Ingredients

- 1 14-ounce can pumpkin puree (about 1 1/2 cups worth)
- 1 ripe banana, mashed
- 1/4 cup coconut flour
- 2/3 cup shredded unsweetened coconut
- 2/3 cup water
- 1 cup full fat coconut milk (this is my favorite brand)
- Pinch of salt
- 2 teaspoons ground cinnamon
- 1 teaspoon ground ginger
- 1/8 teaspoon ground cloves
- 1 teaspoon vanilla extract

- Blueberries, coconut flakes, maple syrup, and/or coconut milk, for serving

Instructions

- Combine the pumpkin puree, banana, coconut flour, shredded coconut, water, coconut milk, salt, cinnamon, ginger, and cloves in a medium size saucepan over low heat.
- Bring to a simmer, stirring constantly, until the mixture is thickened to the consistency of oatmeal. Remove from heat and stir in vanilla extract.
- Spoon into serving bowls and top with blueberries, coconut flakes, maple syrup, coconut milk— whatever makes you happy!

AIP Garlic-Roasted Brussels Sprouts Recipe

INGREDIENTS

- 16 Brussels sprouts (11oz or 320 g)
- 5 cloves of garlic (15 g), unpeeled
- 3 Tablespoons of olive oil (45 ml)
- salt
- zest of 1 lemon

INSTRUCTIONS

- Preheat the oven to 350°F (180°C).
- Slice the Brussels sprouts in half and place in a bowl with the unpeeled garlic cloves. Add the olive oil and toss well to coat.
- Spread on a baking tray and bake in the oven for 25 minutes. Remove

tray and pick out the garlic cloves. Set the sprouts aside to keep warm.

- Squeeze the soft pulp out of the garlic cloves then mix in with the warm Brussels sprouts. Season with salt and serve with finely grated lemon zest.

White Chicken AIP Chili

Ingredients

- 1 onion
- 2 celery stalks
- 4 garlic cloves
- 1 tbsp coconut oil
- 1.5 lbs boneless chicken thighs or breasts
- 1 tsp dried oregano
- 1 tsp onion powder

- 1 tsp garlic powder
- 1 tsp salt
- 4 cups bone broth
- 2 limes
- 1 14-oz can of full-fat coconut milk
- Optional: cilantro, green onion, plantain chips, avocado for garnishment

Instructions

- Dice onion, chop celery, and mince garlic cloves.
- Heat coconut oil over medium-high heat. Add onion, celery, and garlic and cook stirring for 5 minutes.
- Push the veggies to the side then add the chicken.
- Season with dried oregano, onion powder, garlic powder, and salt.

- Cook for 5 minutes, until chicken is browned on all sides.
- Add the bone broth to the pot and squeeze in juice from limes, and bring to boil.
- Lower heat to medium-low, and simmer for 10 minutes.
- Remove chicken and transfer to a bowl, then use 2 forks to shred it completely.
- Add the chicken back to soup, then add coconut milk.
- Increase heat to medium-high, then boil for 10 minutes until the soup is slightly reduced and thickened.
- Garnish as desired.

Hot chocolate

Ingredients

- 1.5 cups boiling water
- 1/2 cup coconut milk
- 1 tbsp carob powder
- 2 tbsp maple flakes
- 1 tbsp gelatin or collagen
- 1 tsp vanilla extract (*for strict AIP use 1/2 tsp vanilla bean powder OR omit all together)
- pinch salt

Instructions

- Add all ingredients to blender.
- Purée.
- Enjoy!

Olive Salad

Ingredients

- 3 whole green onion, chopped
- 1/2 whole red onion, chopped
- 1 cup artichoke hearts, chopped
- 3 ounces black olive, sliced
- 3 ounces kalamata olives, sliced
- 3 ounces green olive, sliced
- 1/4 cup apple cider vinegar
- 1/4 cup extra virgin olive oil
- 1 teaspoon dried oregano
- 1 teaspoon dried parsley
- 1 teaspoon dried basil
- 1/2 teaspoon ground ginger
- 1/2 teaspoon garlic powder

Instructions

- Combine all ingredients and marinade in the fridge for at least 30 minutes before serving.

Paleo Orange Beef Stir Fry

INGREDIENTS

- ó lb (225 g) beef round, sliced into thin slices (1-inch in length)
- 2 small oranges, chopped
- 2 cloves garlic, minced
- 1 teaspoon freshly grated ginger (optional)
- 2 tablespoons (30 ml) tamari sauce (use coconut aminos for AIP) (find tamari here and coconut aminos here)

- 2 tablespoons chopped green onions (scallions)
- 1 tablespoon (15 ml) coconut oil or avocado oil to cook in (find raw, organic coconut oil in bulk here)
- 1 tablespoon cilantro, chopped (for garnish)
- Salt to taste

INSTRUCTIONS

- Place the coconut or avocado oil into a skillet, wok or frying pan. Add in the scallions and then the beef slices and sauté on high heat until most of the beef has turned brown.
- Add in the oranges, garlic, ginger and tamari sauce and sauté on high for 2-3 minutes more until the beef is fully cooked.

- Add salt to taste, garnish with
  cilantro, and serve.

Aip paleo bone broth cabbage detox soup

Ingredients

- 2 tablespoons coconut oil
- 4 cups thinly sliced Savoy cabbage
  about 1/2 of a small head
- 1 medium yellow onion halved and
  thinly sliced
- 1 medium carrot thinly sliced into
  circles
- 4 cloves garlic crushed or minced
- 1 tablespoon fresh-grated ginger
- 3 cups chicken bone broth
- 1 tablespoon coconut aminos
- 1/2 teaspoon ground turmeric

- 1/4 teaspoon sea salt
- 1/4 teaspoon black pepper
- 1 tablespoon chicken bone broth collagen I use Vital Proteins
- 1 tablespoon apple cider vinegar
- 1/2 cup chopped fresh cilantro or scallion

Instructions

- Heat the oil in a medium pot over medium-high heat. Add the cabbage, onion, and carrot, and cook until the vegetables are starting to soften and slightly caramelize in places, about 4 to 5 minutes, stirring frequently.
- Turn the heat down to medium, add the garlic and ginger, and cook 1 minute, stirring constantly.
- Add the broth, coconut aminos, turmeric, salt, and black pepper.

Bring up to a boil, and then cover the pot and simmer until the vegetables are tender, about 5 minutes.

- Turn off the heat. Stir in the chicken bone broth collagen until dissolved, and then stir in the vinegar and cilantro or scallion.
- Serve.

SWEET POTATO CHICKEN POPPERS

INGREDIENTS

- 1 lb ground chicken (uncooked)
- 2 cups uncooked sweet potato, finely grated (I used a wide cheese grater like this or you can use your food processor)
- 2 tbsp coconut oil + 1 tsp for greasing the baking sheet

- 2 tbsp coconut flour (I recommend this brand)
- 2–3 sprigs green onion, chopped fine
- 1 tbsp garlic powder
- 1 tbsp onion powder
- 1 tsp sea salt
- 1/2 tsp black pepper (omit for AIP)
- Optional: 1 tsp paprika or chili powder (not AIP but adds a kick!)

INSTRUCTIONS

- Preheat the oven to 400 F and line a baking sheet with parchment paper lightly greased with oil
- Combine all of the ingredients in a large mixing bowl and thoroughly mix.
- Begin rolling the mixture into small, slightly flattened poppers about one inch in diameter (you'll have about

20-25 poppers) and place them on the baking sheet
- Place in the oven for 25-28 minutes, flipping halfway through. Crisp further in a pan or place under the broiler if desired for 1-2 minutes to crisp further. Remove from the oven when thoroughly cooked through
- Allow to cool and serve with your favorite sauce! These are made for dipping so pair them with guacamole, ketchup, mustard, etc!

AIP Paleo Mediterranean Chicken

Ingredients

- 5-6 Organic Chicken Thighs
- 2-3 Tbs EVOO
- 1 onion chopped

- 2-3 cloves garlic, minced
- 1/2 c. kalamata olives
- 1/4 c. capers
- 1 bag of frozen artichokes or 1 jar
- 1 tsp oregano
- 2 Tbs fresh basil - optional
- 2 handfuls of fresh spinach- optional
- sea salt to taste

Instructions

- Preheat oven to 375*
- Add EVOO or fat of choice to the casserole dish.
- Salt Chicken on both sides
- Add onions, garlic, olives, capers, artichokes, oregano, basil & spinach to the casserole dish.
- Add Chicken on top.

- Bake for 30-40 min or until chicken is done. Juices should be clear. Turn chicken halfway through cooking.

Notes

- If you can't find artichokes without citric acid (they are hard to find) soak them in water with a couple of Tbs. of vinegar & rinse a couple of times thoroughly. I don't know if this removes it totally, but it makes me feel better.
- If you like you can add basil & spinach, stir, & Bake for another 5 min until wilted.

Sweet Potato Breakfast Hash Recipe

Ingredients

- 1 Onion
- 2-3 Garlic Cloves
- 1 Large Sweet Potato
- 1/2 to 1 Head of Broccoli
- 1-2 Apples
- Salt
- Coconut Oil, for frying
- 1 Tablespoon Extra Virgin Olive Oil (Optional)

Instructions

- Heat the coconut oil over medium to high heat in a frying pan.
- Peel and chop the onion and garlic and add to the frying pan, when hot.

- Chop the ends off of the sweet potato, peel and dice into bite sized pieces.
- Add the sweet potato to the frying pan, along with a couple of shakes of salt.
- Chop the broccoli into bite sized pieces and add to the frying pan.
- Peel and chop the apple into small pieces and add to the frying pan.
- Add salt to taste, more coconut oil when needed and cook until all the vegetables have softened and browned to your liking.
- Just before the breakfast hash is ready, you can drizzle over the optional tablespoon of extra virgin olive oil, for extra flavour, nutrition and healthy fats.